Mediterr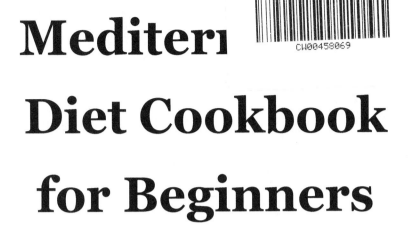 Diet Cookbook for Beginners

50 Healthy Recipes Perfect for Busy and Novice People

By Lucy Richards

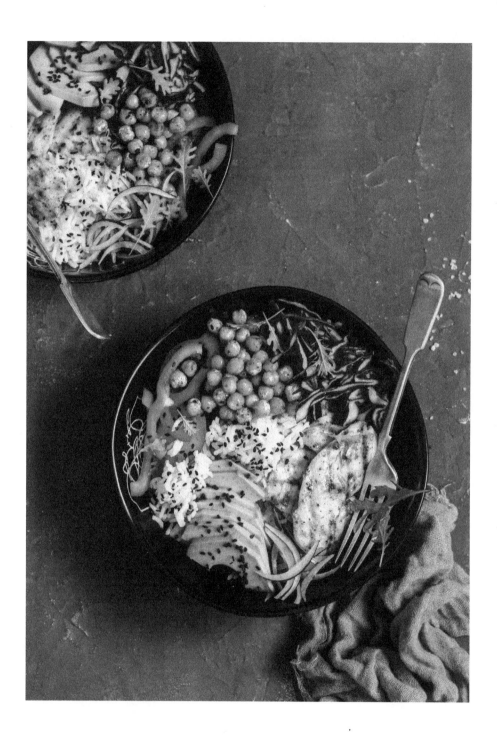

Table of Contents

Chapter 7: Dessert Recipes 100

Introduction

Mediterranean diet is based on the eating habits of the inhabitants of the regions along the Mediterranean Sea, mostly from Italy, Spain and Greece; it is considered more a life style then a diet, in fact it also promotes physical activity and proper liquid (mostly water) consumption.

Depending on fresh seasonal local foods there are no strict rules, because of the many cultural differences, but there are some common factors.

Mediterranean diet has become famous for its ability to reduce heart disease and obesity, thanks to the low consumption of unhealthy fats that increase blood glucose.

Mediterranean diet is mostly plant based, so it's rich of antioxidants; vegetables, fruits like apple and grapes, olive oil, whole grains, herbs, beans and nuts are consumed in large quantities.

Moderate amounts of poultry, eggs, dairy and seafood are also common aliments, accompanied by a little bit of red wine (some studies say that in small amount it helps to stay healthy).

Red meat and sweets like cookies and cakes are accepted but are more limited in quantity.

Foods to avoid:

- refined grains, such as white bread and pasta
- dough containing white flour refined oils (even canola oil and soybean oil)
- foods with added sugars (like pastries, sodas, and candies)
- processed meats processed or packaged foods

Chapter 1: Breakfast and Snack Recipes

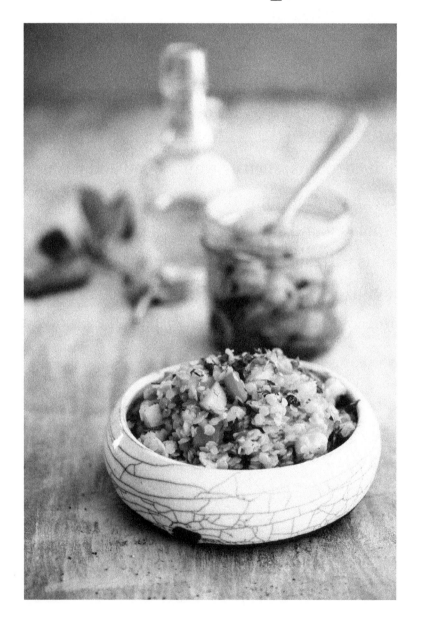

Ham Spinach Ballet

Servings: 2 | Cooking: 40 min

Ingredients

- 4 teaspoons cream
- ¾ pound fresh baby spinach
- 7-ounce ham, sliced
- Salt and black pepper, to taste
- 1 tablespoon unsalted butter, melted

Directions:

1. Preheat the oven to 360 degrees F. and grease 2 ramekins with butter.
2. Put butter and spinach in a skillet and cook for about 3 minutes.
3. Add cooked spinach in the ramekins and top with ham slices, cream, salt and black pepper.
4. Bake for about 25 minutes and dish out to serve hot.
5. For meal prepping, you can refrigerate this ham spinach ballet for about 3 days wrapped in a foil.

Nutrition: Calories: 188 Fat: 12.5g Carbohydrates: 4.9g Protein: 14.6g Sugar: 0.3g Sodium: 1098mg

Banana Quinoa

Servings: 4 | Cooking: 12 min

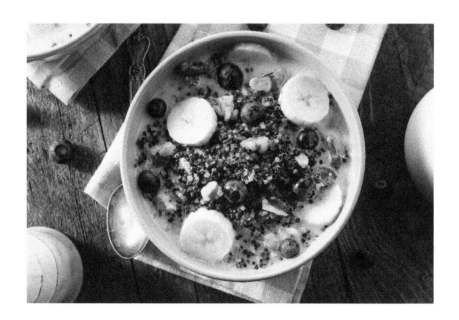

Ingredients

- 1 cup quinoa
- 2 cup milk
- 1 teaspoon vanilla extract
- 1 teaspoon honey
- 2 bananas, sliced
- ¼ teaspoon ground cinnamon

Directions

1. Pour milk in the saucepan and add quinoa.
2. Close the lid and cook it over the medium heat for 12 minutes or until quinoa will absorb all liquid.
3. Then chill the quinoa for 10-15 minutes and place in the serving mason jars.
4. Add honey, vanilla extract, and ground cinnamon.
5. Stir well.
6. Top quinoa with banana and stir it before serving.

Nutrition: Calories 279; fat 5.3; fiber 4.6; carbs 48.4; protein 10.7

Cheesy Eggs Ramekins

Servings: 2 | Cooking: 10 min

Ingredients

- 1 tablespoon chives, chopped
- 1 tablespoon dill, chopped
- A pinch of salt and black pepper
- 2 tablespoons cheddar cheese, grated
- 1 tomato, chopped
- 2 eggs, whisked
- Cooking: spray

Directions

1. In a bowl, mix the eggs with the tomato and the rest of the ingredients except the cooking spray and whisk well.
2. Grease 2 ramekins with the cooking spray, divide the mix into each ramekin, bake at 400 degrees F for 10 minutes and serve.

Nutrition: calories 104; fat 7.1; fiber 0.6; carbs 2.6; protein 7.9

Mediterranean Frittata

Servings: 6 | Cooking: 15 min

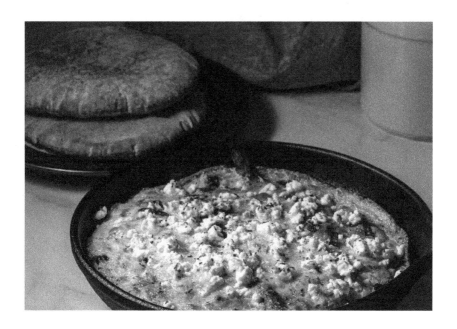

Ingredients

- 8 eggs
- 3 tablespoons olive oil, divided
- 2 tablespoons Parmesan cheese, finely shredded
- 1/8 teaspoon ground black pepper
- 1/4 cup low-fat milk
- 1/4 cup fresh basil, slivered
- 1/2 of a 7-ounce jar (about 1/2 cup) roasted red sweet peppers, drained, chopped

- 1/2 cup onion-and-garlic croutons, purchased, coarsely crushed
- 1/2 cup kalamata or ripe olives, sliced, pitted
- 1/2 cup (2 ounces) feta cheese, crumbled
- 1 teaspoon garlic, bottled minced
- 1 cup onion, chopped

Directions

1. Preheat broiler.
2. In a cast-iron skillet over medium heat, heat 2 tablespoons of the olive oil. Add the garlic and the onion; cook until the onions are just tender.
3. In a large bowl, combine the eggs and the milk; beat. Stir in the feta, sweet peppers, basil, olives, and black pepper. Pour the egg mixture into the skillet and cook. As the mixture sets, using a spatula, lift the egg mixture to allow the uncooked liquid to flow underneath. Continue cooking and lifting until the egg is almost set but the surface is still moist. Reduce the heat, if necessary, to prevent overcooking.

4. In a small-sized bowl, combine the parmesan, croutons, and the remaining 1 tablespoon of olive oil; sprinkle the mixture over the frittata.
5. Transfer the skillet under the broiler about 4-5 inches from the source of heat; broil for about 1-2 minutes, or until the top is set.

Nutrition:242 Cal, 19 g total fat (6 g sat. fat), 297 mg chol., 339 mg sodium, 7g carb.,1 g fiber,12 g protein.

Cinnamon Apple And Lentils Porridge

Servings: 4 | Cooking: 10 min

Ingredients

- ½ cup walnuts, chopped
- 2 green apples, cored, peeled and cubed
- 3 tablespoons maple syrup
- 3 cups almond milk
- ½ cup red lentils
- ½ teaspoon cinnamon powder
- ½ cup cranberries, dried
- 1 teaspoon vanilla extract

Directions

1. Put the milk in a pot, heat it up over medium heat, add the walnuts, apples, maple syrup and the rest of the ingredients, toss, simmer for 10 minutes, divide into bowls and serve.

Nutrition: calories 150; fat 2; fiber 1; carbs 3; protein 5

Creamy Oatmeal

Servings: 2 | Cooking: 15 min

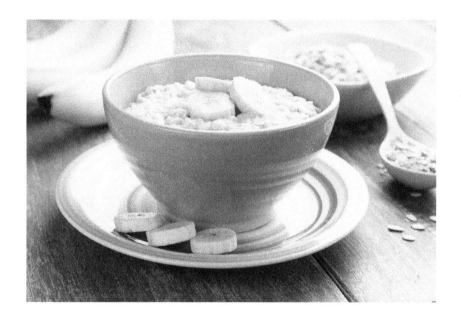

Ingredients

- 1 ½ cup oatmeal
- 1 tablespoon cocoa powder
- ½ cup heavy cream
- ¼ cup of water
- 1 teaspoon vanilla extract
- 1 tablespoon butter
- 2 tablespoons Splenda

Directions

1. Mix up together oatmeal with cocoa powder and Splenda.
2. Transfer the mixture in the saucepan.
3. Add vanilla extract, water, and heavy cream. Stir it gently with the help of the spatula.
4. Close the lid and cook it for 10-15 minutes over the medium-low heat.
5. Remove the cooked cocoa oatmeal from the heat and add butter. Stir it well.

Nutrition: calories 230; fat 10.6; fiber 3.5; carbs 28.1; protein 4.6

Stuffed Sweet Potato

Servings: 8 | Cooking: 40 min

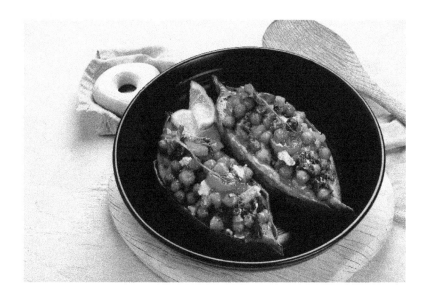

Ingredients

- 8 sweet potatoes, pierced with a fork
- 14 ounces canned chickpeas, drained and rinsed
- 1 small red bell pepper, chopped
- 1 tablespoon lemon zest, grated
- 2 tablespoons lemon juice
- 3 tablespoons olive oil
- 1 teaspoon garlic, minced
- 1 tablespoon oregano, chopped
- 2 tablespoons parsley, chopped

- A pinch of salt and black pepper
- 1 avocado, peeled, pitted and mashed
- ¼ cup water
- ¼ cup tahini paste

Directions

1. Arrange the potatoes on a baking sheet lined with parchment paper, bake them at 400 degrees F for 40 minutes, cool them down and cut a slit down the middle in each.
2. In a bowl, combine the chickpeas with the bell pepper, lemon zest, half of the lemon juice, half of the oil, half of the garlic, oregano, half of the parsley, salt and pepper, toss and stuff the potatoes with this mix.
3. In another bowl, mix the avocado with the water, tahini, the rest of the lemon juice, oil, garlic and parsley, whisk well and spread over the potatoes.
4. Serve cold for breakfast.

Nutrition: calories 308; fat 2; fiber 8; carbs 38; protein 7

Couscous And Chickpeas Bowls

Servings: 4 | Cooking: 6 min

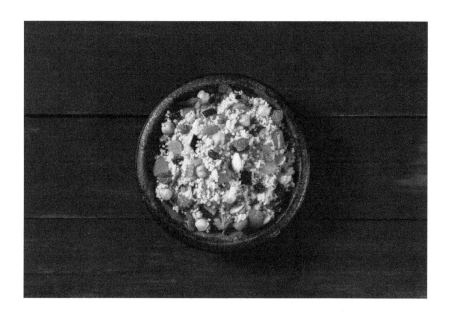

Ingredients

- ¾ cup whole wheat couscous
- 1 yellow onion, chopped
- 1 tablespoon olive oil
- 1 cup water
- 2 garlic cloves, minced
- 15 ounces canned chickpeas, drained and rinsed
- A pinch of salt and black pepper
- 15 ounces canned tomatoes, chopped

- 14 ounces canned artichokes, drained and chopped
- ½ cup Greek olives, pitted and chopped
- ½ teaspoon oregano, dried
- 1 tablespoon lemon juice

Directions

1. Put the water in a pot, bring to a boil over medium heat, add the couscous, stir, take off the heat, cover the pan, leave aside for 10 minutes and fluff with a fork.
2. Heat up a pan with the oil over medium-high heat, add the onion and sauté for 2 minutes.
3. Add the rest of the ingredients, toss and cook for 4 minutes more.
4. Add the couscous, toss, divide into bowls and serve for breakfast.

Nutrition: calories 340; fat 10; fiber 9; carbs 51; protein 11

Vegetarian Three Cheese Quiche Stuffed Peppers

Servings: 2 | Cooking: 50 min

Ingredients:

- 2 large eggs
- ¼ cup mozzarella, shredded
- 1 medium bell peppers, sliced in half and seeds removed
- ¼ cup ricotta cheese
- ¼ cup grated Parmesan cheese
- ½ teaspoon garlic powder
- 1/8 cup baby spinach leaves
- ¼ teaspoon dried parsley
- 1 tablespoon Parmesan cheese, to garnish

Directions

1. Preheat oven to 375 degrees F.
2. Blend all the cheeses, eggs, garlic powder and parsley in a food processor and process until smooth.

3. Pour the cheese mixture into each sliced bell pepper and top with spinach leaves.
4. Stir with a fork, pushing them under the cheese mixture and cover with foil.
5. Bake for about 40 minutes and sprinkle with Parmesan cheese.
6. Broil for about 5 minutes and dish out to serve.

Nutrition: Calories: 157 Carbs: 7.3g Fats: 9g Proteins: 12.7g Sodium: 166mg Sugar: 3.7g

Sweet Bread With Dates

Servings: 1 Roll | Cooking: 30 min

Ingredients:

- 23/4 cups all-purpose flour
- 1/4 cup dry milk
- 1/4 cup sugar
- 11/4 tsp. salt
- 1 TB. instant yeast
- 3 large eggs
- 1/3 cup plus 1 TB. water
- 10 TB. butter
- 12 medjool dates, pitted
- 1 TB. orange blossom water
- 1/2 tsp. cinnamon
- 1 large egg white

Directions

1. In a food processor fitted with a dough attachment or in a blender, knead all-purpose flour, dry milk, sugar, salt, instant yeast, eggs, 1/3 cup water, and 8 tablespoons butter for 15 minutes.

2. Transfer dough to a bowl lightly sprayed with olive oil spray, cover the bowl with plastic wrap, and let rise in the refrigerator for 24 hours.

3. In a food processor fitted with a chopping blade, blend medjool dates, orange blossom water, and cinnamon for 2 minutes or until smooth.

4. Grease a 12-cup muffin tin with remaining 2 tablespoons butter.

5. Form dough into 12 equal pieces. Spoon 1 tablespoon date mixture into center of each dough piece, tightly seal dough around date mixture, and place seal side down into the prepared muffin tin.

6. Set aside dough to rise for 1 hour.

7. Preheat the oven to 375°F.

8. In a small bowl, whisk together egg white and remaining 1 tablespoon water. Brush each roll with egg wash.

9. Bake for 30 minutes.

10. Remove rolls from the oven, and let rest for 20 minutes before serving.

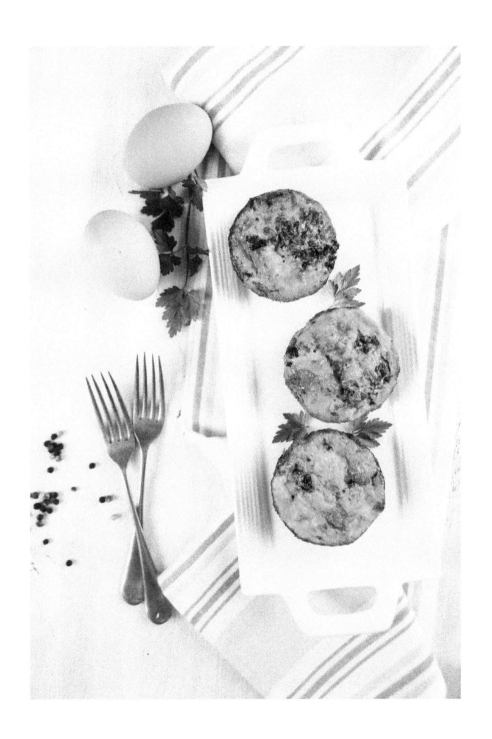

Chapter 2: Lunch & Dinner Recipes

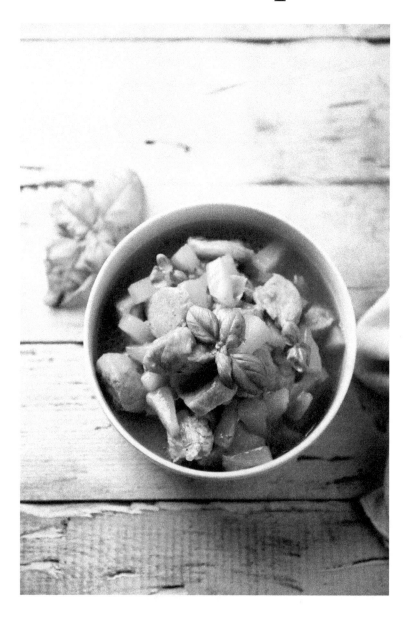

Salmon Parmesan Gratin

Servings: 4 | Cooking: 45 min

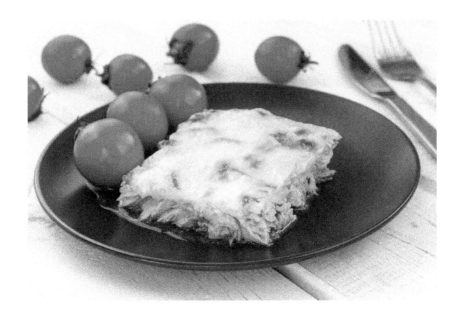

Ingredients

- 4 salmon fillets, cubed
- 2 garlic cloves, chopped
- 1 fennel bulb, sliced
- ½ teaspoon ground coriander
- ½ teaspoon Dijon mustard
- ½ cup vegetable stock
- 1 cup heavy cream
- 2 eggs

- Salt and pepper to taste
- 1 cup grated Parmesan cheese

Directions

1. Combine the salmon, garlic, fennel, coriander and mustard in a small deep dish baking pan.
2. Mix the eggs with cream and stock and pour the mixture over the fish.
3. Top with Parmesan cheese and bake in the preheated oven at 350F for 25 minutes.
4. Serve the gratin right away.

Nutrition: Calories:414 Fat:25.9g Protein:41.0g Carbohydrates:6.1g

Sweet And Sour Chicken Fillets

Servings: 4 | Cooking: 40 min

Ingredients

- 4 chicken fillets
- 3 tablespoons olive oil
- 1 red pepper, sliced
- 1 lemon, juiced
- 1 tablespoon honey
- Salt and pepper to taste
- Chopped parsley for serving

Directions

1. Season the chicken with salt and pepper.
2. Heat the oil in a skillet and add the chicken.
3. Cook on each side for 10 minutes.
4. Add the red pepper, lemon juice and honey and cook just for 1 additional minute.
5. Serve the chicken and the sauce warm and fresh.

Nutrition: Calories:309 Fat:18.0g Protein:29.4g Carbohydrates:7.5g

Salt Crusted Salmon

Servings: 6 | Cooking: 40 min

Ingredients

- 1 whole salmon (3 pounds)
- 3 cups salt
- ½ cup chopped parsley
- 3 tablespoons olive oil

Directions

1. Spread a very thin layer of salt in a baking tray.
2. Place the salmon over the salt and top with parsley. Drizzle with oil then top with the rest of the salt.
3. Cook in the preheated oven at 350F for 30 minutes.
4. Serve the salmon warm.

Nutrition: Calories:362 Fat:21.0g Protein:44.1g Carbohydrates:0.3g

Sun-dried Tomato Pesto Penne

Servings: 4 | Cooking: 20 min

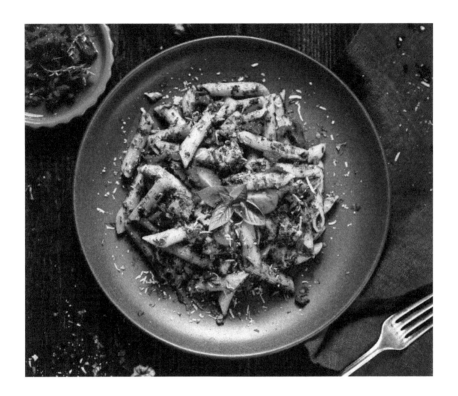

Ingredients

- 8 oz. penne
- ½ cup sun-dried tomatoes, drained well
- 2 tablespoons olive oil
- 4 garlic cloves, minced
- 2 tablespoons lemon juice
- 2 tablespoons pine nuts

- 2 tablespoons grated Parmesan cheese
- 1 pinch chili flakes

Directions

1. Cook the penne in a large pot of salty water for 8 minutes or as long as it says on the package, just until al dente.
2. Drain the penne well.
3. For the pesto, combine the remaining ingredients in a blender and pulse until well mixed and smooth.
4. Mix the pesto with the penne and serve right away.

Nutrition: Calories:308 Fat:14.4g Protein:11.9g Carbohydrates:34.1g

Herbed Marinated Sardines

Servings: 4 | Cooking: 50 min

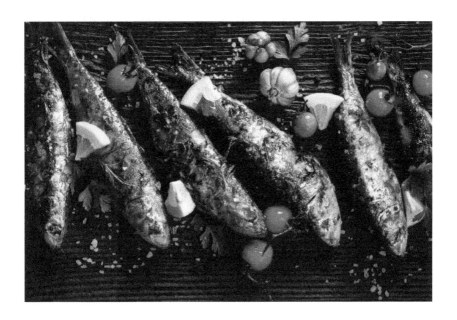

Ingredients

- 8 sardines
- ½ cup chopped parsley
- 2 tablespoons chopped cilantro
- 2 tablespoons pesto sauce
- 2 tablespoons olive oil
- 2 garlic cloves
- Salt and pepper to taste
- 2 tablespoons lemon juice

Directions

1. Combine the herbs, pesto, oil, garlic, salt and pepper in a blender and pulse until smooth.
2. Spread the herb mixture over the sardines and season with salt and pepper.
3. Place the sardines in the fridge for 30 minutes.
4. Heat a grill pan over medium flame and place the sardines on the grill.
5. Cook on each side for 5-7 minutes.
6. Serve the sardines warm and fresh with your favorite side dish.

Nutrition: Calories:201 Fat:15.9g Protein:13.0g Carbohydrates:1.7g

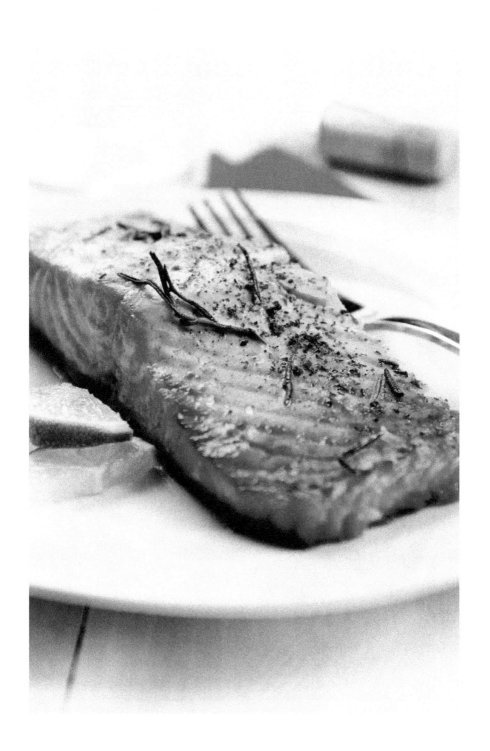

Chapter 3: Meat Recipes

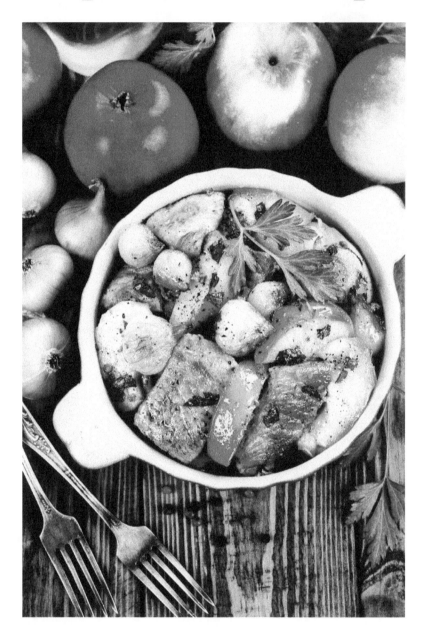

Ita Sandwiches

Servings: 1 Pita Sandwich | Cooking: 20 min

Ingredients

- 1 lb. ground beef
- 1 tsp. salt
- 1/2 tsp. ground black pepper
- 1 tsp. seven spices
- 4 (6- or 7-in.) pitas

Directions

1. Preheat the oven to 400°F.
2. In a medium bowl, combine beef, salt, black pepper, and seven spices.
3. Lay out pitas on the counter, and divide beef mixture evenly among them, and spread beef to edge of pitas.
4. Place pitas on a baking sheet, and bake for 20 minutes.
5. Serve warm with Greek yogurt.

Easy Chicken With Capers Skillet

Servings: 4 | Cooking: 35 min

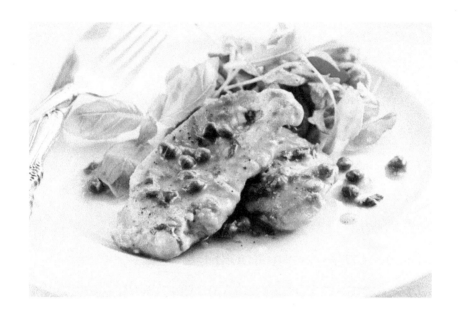

Ingredients

- 4 boneless skinless chicken breast halves (6 ounces each)
- 1/4 teaspoon salt
- 1/4 teaspoon pepper
- 3 tablespoons olive oil
- 1-pint grape tomatoes
- 16 pitted Greek or ripe olives, sliced
- 3 tablespoons capers, drained

Directions

1. Place a cast iron skillet on medium high fire and heat for 5 minutes.
2. Meanwhile, season chicken with pepper and salt.
3. Add oil to pan and heat for another minute. Add chicken and increase fire to high. Brown sides for 4 minutes per side.
4. Lower fire to medium and add capers and tomatoes.
5. Bake uncovered in a 4750F preheated oven for 12 minutes.
6. Remove from oven and let it sit for 5 minutes before serving.

Nutrition: Calories: 336; Carbs: 6.0g; Protein: 36.0g; Fats: 18.0g

Lamb And Dill Apples

Servings: 4 | Cooking: 25 min

Ingredients

- 3 green apples, cored, peeled and cubed
- Juice of 1 lemon
- 1 pound lamb stew meat, cubed
- 1 small bunch dill, chopped
- 3 ounces heavy cream
- 2 tablespoon olive oil
- Salt and black pepper to the taste

Directions

1. Heat up a pan with the oil over medium-high heat, add the lamb and brown for 5 minutes.
2. Add the rest of the ingredients, bring to a simmer and cook over medium heat for 20 minutes.
3. Divide the mix between plates and serve.

Nutrition: calories 328; fat 16.7; fiber 10.5; carbs 21.6; protein 14.7

Tomatoes And Carrots Pork Mix

Servings: 4 | Cooking: 7 Hours

Ingredients

- 2 tablespoons olive oil
- ½ cup chicken stock
- 1 tablespoon ginger, grated
- Salt and black pepper to the taste
- 2 and ½ pounds pork stew meat, roughly cubed
- 2 cups tomatoes, chopped
- 4 ounces carrots, chopped
- 1 tablespoon cilantro, chopped

Directions

1. In your slow cooker, combine the oil with the stock, ginger and the rest of the ingredients, put the lid on and cook on Low for 7 hours.
2. Divide the mix between plates and serve.

Nutrition: calories 303; fat 15; fiber 8.6; carbs 14.9; protein 10.8

Cherry Stuffed Lamb

Servings: 2 | Cooking: 40 min

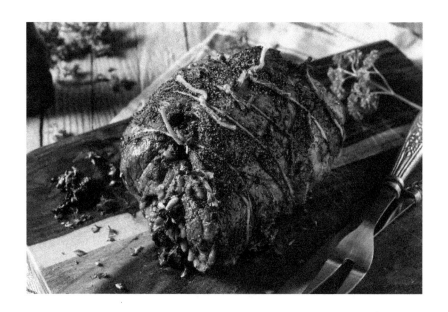

Ingredients

- 9 oz lamb loin
- 1 oz pistachio, chopped
- 1 teaspoon cherries, pitted
- ½ teaspoon olive oil
- ¼ teaspoon dried thyme
- 1 teaspoon dried rosemary
- 1 garlic clove, minced
- ¼ teaspoon liquid honey

Directions

1. Rub the lamb loin with dried thyme and rosemary.
2. Then make a lengthwise cut in the meat.
3. Mix up together pistachios, minced garlic, and cherries.
4. Fill the meat with this mixture and secure the cut with the toothpick.
5. Then brush the lamb loin with liquid honey and olive oil.
6. Wrap the meat in the foil and bake at 365F for 40 minutes.
7. When the meat is cooked, remove it from the foil.
8. Let the meat chill for 10 minutes and then slice it.

Nutrition: calories 353; fat 20.4; fiber 1.8; carbs 6; protein 36.9

Chapter 4: Poultry Recipes

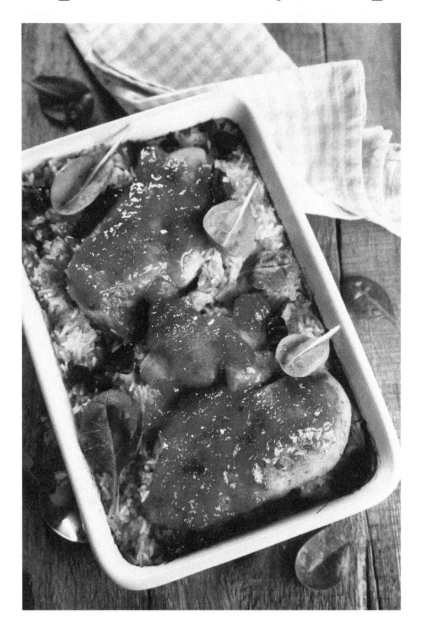

Coriander And Coconut Chicken

Servings: 4 | Cooking: 30 min

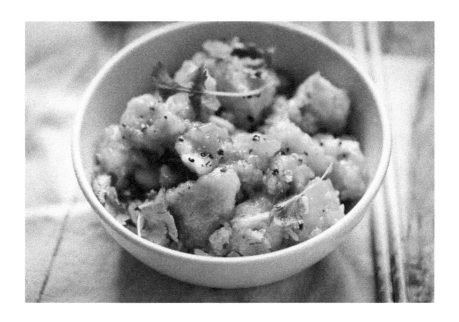

Ingredients

- 2 pounds chicken thighs, skinless, boneless and cubed
- 2 tablespoons olive oil
- Salt and black pepper to the taste
- 3 tablespoons coconut flesh, shredded
- 1 and ½ teaspoons orange extract
- 1 tablespoon ginger, grated
- ¼ cup orange juice

- 2 tablespoons coriander, chopped
- 1 cup chicken stock
- ¼ teaspoon red pepper flakes

Directions

1. Heat up a pan with the oil over medium-high heat, add the chicken and brown for 4 minutes on each side.
2. Add salt, pepper and the rest of the ingredients, bring to a simmer and cook over medium heat for 20 minutes.
3. Divide the mix between plates and serve hot.

Nutrition: calories 297; fat 14.4; fiber 9.6; carbs 22; protein 25

Chicken Pilaf

Servings: 4 | Cooking: 30 min

Ingredients

- 4 tablespoons avocado oil
- 2 pounds chicken breasts, skinless, boneless and cubed
- ½ cup yellow onion, chopped
- 4 garlic cloves, minced
- 8 ounces brown rice
- 4 cups chicken stock
- ½ cup kalamata olives, pitted
- ½ cup tomatoes, cubed
- 6 ounces baby spinach
- ½ cup feta cheese, crumbled
- A pinch of salt and black pepper
- 1 tablespoon marjoram, chopped
- 1 tablespoon basil, chopped
- Juice of ½ lemon
- ¼ cup pine nuts, toasted

Directions

1. Heat up a pot with 1 tablespoon avocado oil over medium-high heat, add the chicken, some salt and pepper, brown for 5 minutes on each side and transfer to a bowl.
2. Heat up the pot again with the rest of the avocado oil over medium heat, add the onion and garlic and sauté for 3 minutes.
3. Add the rice, the rest of the ingredients except the pine nuts, also return the chicken, toss, bring to a simmer and cook over medium heat for 20 minutes.
4. Divide the mix between plates, top each serving with some pine nuts and serve.

Nutrition: calories 283; fat 12.5; fiber 8.2; carbs 21.5; protein 13.4

Chicken And Black Beans

Servings: 4 | Cooking: 20 min

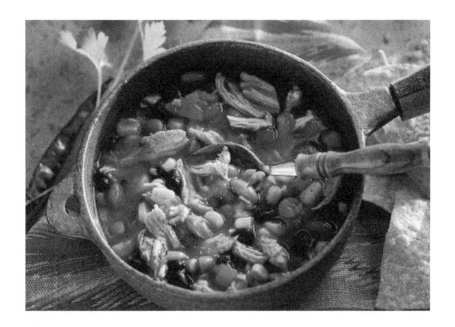

Ingredients

- 12 oz chicken breast, skinless, boneless, chopped
- 1 tablespoon taco seasoning
- 1 tablespoon nut oil
- ½ teaspoon cayenne pepper
- ½ teaspoon salt
- ½ teaspoon garlic, chopped
- ½ red onion, sliced
- 1/3 cup black beans, canned, rinsed

- ½ cup Mozzarella, shredded

Directions

1. Rub the chopped chicken breast with taco seasoning, salt, and cayenne pepper.
2. Place the chicken in the skillet, add nut oil and roast it for 10 minutes over the medium heat. Mix up the chicken pieces from time to time to avoid burning.
3. After this, transfer the chicken in the plate.
4. Add sliced onion and garlic in the skillet. Roast the vegetables for 5 minutes. Stir them constantly. Then add black beans and stir well. Cook the ingredients for 2 minute more.
5. Add the chopped chicken and mix up well. Top the meal with Mozzarella cheese.
6. Close the lid and cook the meal for 3 minutes.

Nutrition: calories 209; fat 6.4; fiber 2.8; carbs 13.7, 22.7

Coconut Chicken

Servings: 4 | Cooking: 5 min

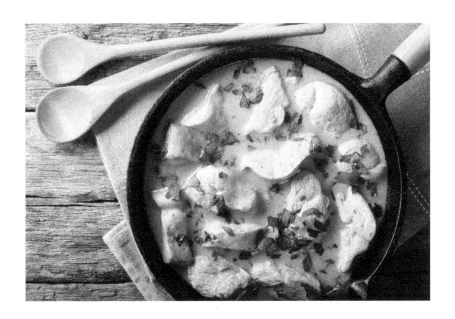

Ingredients

- 6 oz chicken fillet
- ¼ cup of sparkling water
- 1 egg
- 3 tablespoons coconut flakes
- 1 tablespoon coconut oil
- 1 teaspoon Greek Seasoning

Directions

1. Cut the chicken fillet on small pieces (nuggets).

2. Then crack the egg in the bowl and whisk it.
3. Mix up together egg and sparkling water.
4. Add Greek seasoning and stir gently.
5. Dip the chicken nuggets in the egg mixture and then coat in the coconut flakes.
6. Melt the coconut oil in the skillet and heat it up until it is shimmering.
7. Then add prepared chicken nuggets.
8. Roast them for 1 minute from each or until they are light brown.
9. Dry the cooked chicken nuggets with the help of the paper towel and transfer in the serving plates.

Nutrition: calories 141; fat 8.9; fiber 0.3; carbs 1; protein 13.9

Ginger Chicken Drumsticks

Servings: 4 | Cooking: 30 min

Ingredients

- 4 chicken drumsticks
- 1 apple, grated
- 1 tablespoon curry paste
- 4 tablespoons milk
- 1 teaspoon coconut oil
- 1 teaspoon chili flakes
- ½ teaspoon minced ginger

Directions

1. Mix up together grated apple, curry paste, milk, chili flakes, and minced garlic.
2. Put coconut oil in the skillet and melt it.
3. Add apple mixture and stir well.
4. Then add chicken drumsticks and mix up well.
5. Roast the chicken for 2 minutes from each side.
6. Then preheat oven to 360F.
7. Place the skillet with chicken drumsticks in the oven and bake for 25 minutes.

Nutrition: calories 150; fat 6.4; fiber 1.4; carbs 9.7; protein 13.5

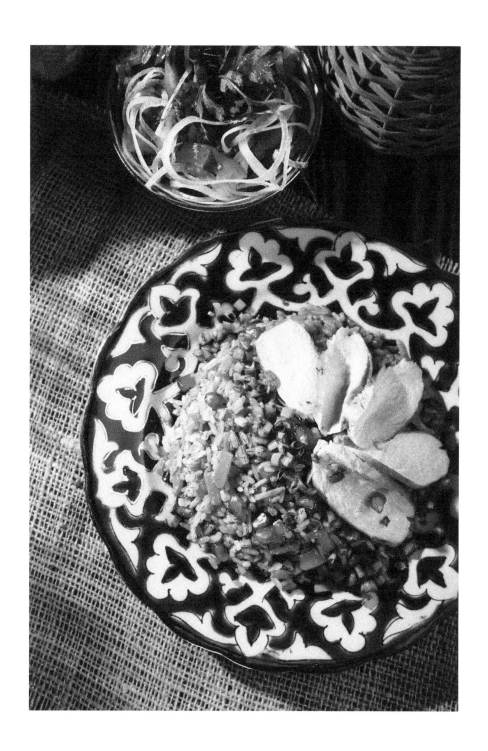

Chapter 5: Fish and Seafood Recipes

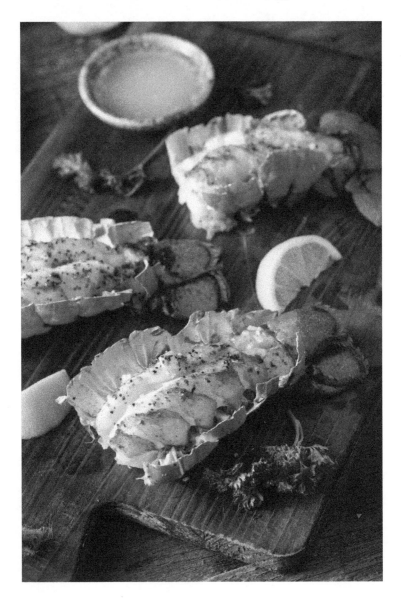

Shrimp Kebabs

Servings: 2 | Cooking: 5 min

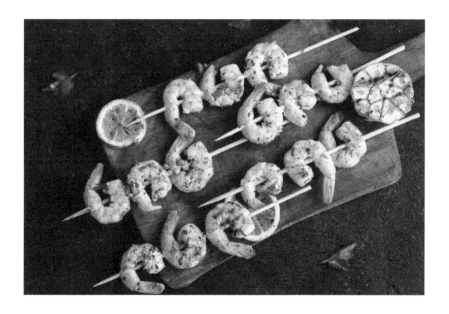

Ingredients

- 4 King prawns, peeled
- 1 tablespoon lemon juice
- ¾ teaspoon ground coriander
- ½ teaspoon salt
- 1 tablespoon tomato sauce
- 1 tablespoon olive oil

Directions

1. Skew the shrimps on the skewers and sprinkle them with lemon juice, ground coriander, salt, and tomato sauce.
2. Then drizzle the shrimps with olive oil.
3. Preheat grill to 385F.
4. Grill the shrimp kebabs for 2 minutes from each side.

Nutrition: calories 106; fat 7.5; fiber 0.4; carbs 0.6; protein 9.1

Easy Broiled Lobster Tails

Servings: 2 | Cooking: 10 min

Ingredients

- 1 6-oz frozen lobster tails
- 1 tbsp olive oil
- 1 tsp lemon pepper seasoning

Directions

1. Preheat oven broiler.
2. With kitchen scissors, cut thawed lobster tails in half lengthwise.
3. Brush with oil the exposed lobster meat. Season with lemon pepper.
4. Place lobster tails in baking sheet with exposed meat facing up.
5. Place on top broiler rack and broil for 10 minutes until lobster meat is lightly browned on the sides and center meat is opaque.
6. Serve and enjoy.

Nutrition: Calories: 175.6; Protein: 3g; Fat: 10g; Carbs: 18.4g

Cajun Garlic Shrimp Noodle Bowl

Servings: 2 | Cooking: 15 min

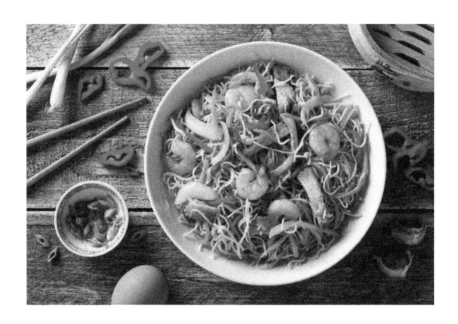

Ingredients

- ½ teaspoon salt
- 1 onion, sliced
- 1 red pepper, sliced
- 1 tablespoon butter
- 1 teaspoon garlic granules
- 1 teaspoon onion powder
- 1 teaspoon paprika
- 2 large zucchinis, cut into noodle strips

- 20 jumbo shrimps, shells removed and deveined
- 3 cloves garlic, minced
- 3 tablespoon ghee
- A dash of cayenne pepper
- A dash of red pepper flakes

Directions

1. Prepare the Cajun seasoning by mixing the onion powder, garlic granules, pepper flakes, cayenne pepper, paprika and salt. Toss in the shrimp to coat in the seasoning.
2. In a skillet, heat the ghee and sauté the garlic. Add in the red pepper and onions and continue sautéing for 4 minutes.
3. Add the Cajun shrimp and cook until opaque. Set aside.
4. In another pan, heat the butter and sauté the zucchini noodles for three minutes.
5. Assemble by the placing the Cajun shrimps on top of the zucchini noodles.

Nutrition: Calories: 712; Fat: 30.0g; Protein: 97.8g; Carbs: 20.2g

Red Peppers & Pineapple Topped Mahi-mahi

Servings: 4 | Cooking: 30 min

Ingredients

- ¼ tsp black pepper
- ¼ tsp salt
- 1 cup whole wheat couscous
- 1 red bell pepper, diced
- 2 1/3 cups low sodium chicken broth
- 2 cups chopped fresh pineapple
- 2 tbsp. chopped fresh chives
- 2 tsp. olive oil
- 4 pieces of skinless, boneless mahi mahi (dolphin fish) fillets (around 4-oz each)

Directions

1. On high fire, add 1 1/3 cups broth to a small saucepan and heat until boiling. Once boiling, add couscous. Turn off fire, cover and set aside to allow liquid to be fully absorbed around 5 minutes.
2. On medium high fire, place a large nonstick saucepan and heat oil.

3. Season fish on both sides with pepper and salt. Add mahi mahi to hot pan and pan fry until golden around one minute each side. Once cooked, transfer to plate.
4. On same pan, sauté bell pepper and pineapples until soft, around 2 minutes on medium high fire.
5. Add couscous to pan along with chives, and remaining broth.
6. On top of the mixture in pan, place fish. With foil, cover pan and continue cooking until fish is steaming and tender underneath the foil, around 3-5 minutes.

Nutrition: Calories per serving: 302; Protein: 43.1g; Fat: 4.8g; Carbs: 22.0g

Dill Halibut

Servings: 3 | Cooking: 10 min

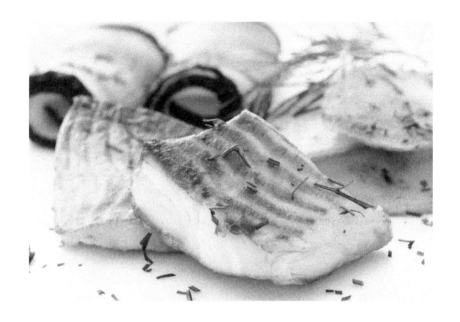

Ingredients

- 13 oz halibut fillet
- 1/3 cup cream
- ¼ cup dill, chopped
- ½ teaspoon garlic powder
- ¼ teaspoon turmeric
- ¼ teaspoon ground paprika
- 1 teaspoon salt
- 1 teaspoon olive oil

Directions

1. Chop the fish fillet on the big cubes and sprinkle them with garlic powder, turmeric, ground paprika, and salt.
2. Pour olive oil in the skillet and preheat it well.
3. Then place fish in the hot oil and roast it for 2 minutes from each side over the medium heat.
4. Add cream and stir gently with the help of the spatula.
5. Bring the mixture to boil and add dill.
6. Close the lid and cook fish on the medium heat for 5 minutes. Till the fish and creamy sauce are cooked.
7. Serve the halibut cubes with creamy sauce.

Nutrition: calories 170; fat 5.9; fiber 0.7; carbs 3.6; protein 25.1

Chapter 6: Salads & Side Dishes

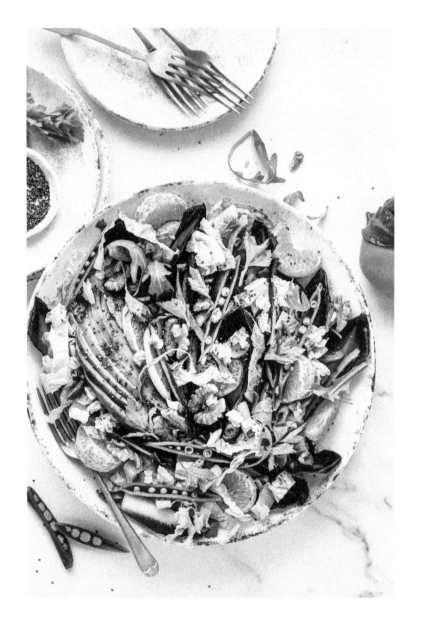

Red Wine Dressed Arugula Salad

Servings: 2 | Cooking: 12 min

Ingredients

- ¼ cup red onion, sliced thinly
- 1 ½ tbsp fresh lemon juice
- 1 ½ tbsp olive oil
- 1 tbsp extra-virgin olive oil
- 1 tbsp red-wine vinegar
- 2 center cut salmon fillets (6-oz each)
- 2/3 cup cherry tomatoes, halved
- 3 cups baby arugula leaves
- Pepper and salt to taste

Directions

1. In a shallow bowl, mix pepper, salt, 1 ½ tbsp olive oil and lemon juice. Toss in salmon fillets and rub with the marinade. Allow to marinate for at least 15 minutes.
2. Grease a baking sheet and preheat oven to 350oF.
3. Bake marinated salmon fillet for 10 to 12 minutes or until flaky with skin side touching the baking sheet.

4. Meanwhile, in a salad bowl mix onion, tomatoes and arugula.
5. Season with pepper and salt. Drizzle with vinegar and oil. Toss to combine and serve right away with baked salmon on the side.

Nutrition: Calories per serving: 400; Protein: 36.6g; Carbs: 5.8g; Fat: 25.6g

Artichoke Farro Salad

Servings: 6 | Cooking: 30 min

Ingredients

- 1 cup faro
- 2 cups vegetable stock
- 6 artichoke hearts, chopped
- ½ cup chopped parsley
- 2 tablespoons chopped cilantro
- 2 garlic cloves, chopped
- 2 tablespoons extra virgin olive oil
- Salt and pepper to taste
- 4 oz. feta cheese, crumbled

Directions

1. Combine the faro and stock in a saucepan and cook on low heat until all the liquid has been absorbed.
2. When done, transfer the faro in a salad bowl then stir in the rest of the ingredients.
3. Adjust the taste with salt and pepper and mix well.
4. Serve the salad fresh.

Nutrition: Calories:171 Fat:9.0g Protein:8.3g
Carbohydrates:18.8g

Balsamic Tomato Mix

Servings: 4 | Cooking: 0 min

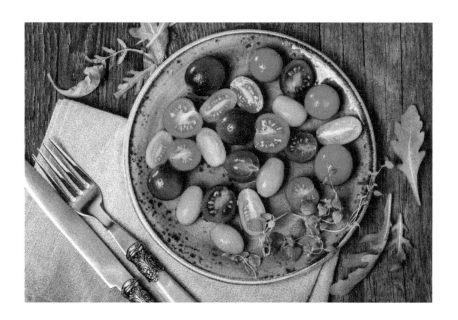

Ingredients

- 2 pounds cherry tomatoes, halved
- 2 tablespoons olive oil
- 2 tablespoons balsamic vinegar
- 1 garlic clove, minced
- 1 cup basil, chopped
- 1 tablespoon chives, chopped
- Salt and black pepper to the taste

Directions

1. In a bowl, combine the tomatoes with the garlic, basil and the rest of the ingredients, toss and serve as a side salad.

Nutrition: calories 200; fat 5.6; fiber 4.5; carbs 15.1; protein 4.3

Gigantes Plaki

Servings: 4 | Cooking: 2 Hour

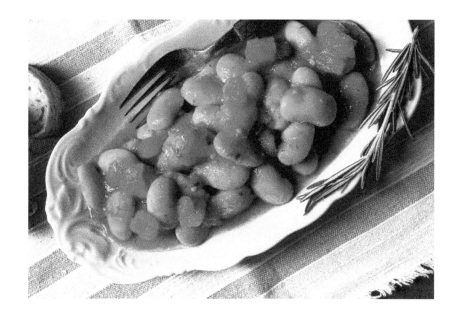

Ingredients

- 1 Spanish onion, finely chopped
- 1 teaspoon dried oregano
- 1 teaspoon sugar
- 2 garlic cloves, finely chopped
- 2 tablespoons flat-leaf parsley, chopped, plus more to serve
- 2 tablespoons tomato purée

- 3 tablespoons extra-virgin olive oil, plus more to serve
- 400 g dried butter beans
- 800 g ripe tomatoes, skinned, roughly chopped
- Pinch ground cinnamon

Directions

1. In water, soak the beans overnight, drain, rinse, and then place in a pan filled with water; bring to a boil. When boiling, reduce the heat to a simmer, cooking for about 50 minutes or until the beans are slightly tender but still not soft. Drain and set aside.
2. Preheat the oven to 180C, gas to 4, or fan to 160C.
3. In a large-sized frying pan, heat the olive oil. Add the onion and the garlic; cook for 10 minutes over medium heat or until soft but not browned.
4. Add the tomato puree, cook for 1 minute more. Add the rest of the ingredients; simmer for about 2 to 3 minutes, season generously, then stir in the beans. Pour the mixture into an oven-safe dish; bake for 1 hour, uncovered, without stirring, or until the beans are tender.

Nutrition:431 cal, 11 g fat (1 g sat. fat), 66 g carbs, 15 g sugars, 19 g fiber, 22 g protein, and 0.2 g sodium.

Squash And Tomatoes Mix

Servings: 6 | Cooking: 20 min

Ingredients

- 5 medium squash, cubed
- A pinch of salt and black pepper
- 3 tablespoons olive oil
- 1 cup pine nuts, toasted
- ¼ cup goat cheese, crumbled
- 6 tomatoes, cubed
- ½ yellow onion, chopped
- 2 tablespoons cilantro, chopped
- 2 tablespoons lemon juice

Directions

1. Heat up a pan with the oil over medium heat, add the onion and pine nuts and cook for 3 minutes.
2. Add the squash and the rest of the ingredients, cook everything for 15 minutes, divide between plates and serve as a side dish.

Nutrition: calories 200; fat 4.5; fiber 3.4; carbs 6.7; protein 4

Chickpeas, Corn And Black Beans Salad

Servings: 4 | Cooking: 0 min

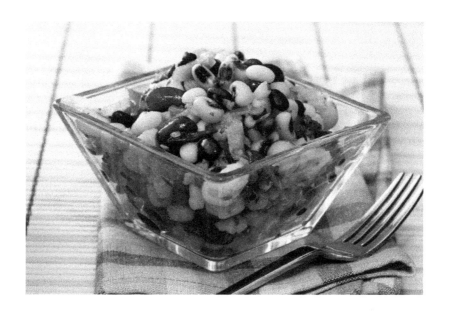

Ingredients

- 1 and ½ cups canned black beans, drained and rinsed
- ½ teaspoon garlic powder
- 2 teaspoons chili powder
- A pinch of sea salt and black pepper
- 1 and ½ cups canned chickpeas, drained and rinsed

- 1 cup baby spinach
- 1 avocado, pitted, peeled and chopped
- 1 cup corn kernels, chopped
- 2 tablespoons lemon juice
- 1 tablespoon olive oil
- 1 tablespoon apple cider vinegar
- 1 teaspoon chives, chopped

Directions

1. In a salad bowl, combine the black beans with the garlic powder, chili powder and the rest of the ingredients, toss and serve cold.

Nutrition: calories 300; fat 13.4; fiber 4.1; carbs 8.6; protein 13

Eggplant And Bell Pepper Mix

Servings: 4 | Cooking: 45 min

Ingredients

- 2 green bell peppers, cut into strips
- 2 eggplants, sliced
- 2 tablespoons tomato paste
- Salt and black pepper to the taste
- 4 garlic cloves, minced
- ¼ cup olive oil
- 1 tablespoon cilantro, chopped
- 1 tablespoon chives, chopped

Directions

1. In a roasting pan, combine the bell peppers with the eggplants and the rest of the ingredients, introduce in the oven and cook at 380 degrees F for 45 minutes.
2. Divide the mix between plates and serve as a side dish.

Nutrition: calories 207; fat 13.3; fiber 10.5; carbs 23.4; protein 3.8

Broccoli Salad With Caramelized Onions

Servings: 4 | Cooking: 25 min

Ingredients

- Extra virgin olive oil - 3 tbsp.
- Red onions - 2, sliced
- Dried thyme - 1 tsp.
- Balsamic vinegar - 2 tbsp. vinegar
- Broccoli - 1 lb., cut into florets
- Salt and pepper - to taste

Directions

1. Heat extra virgin olive oil in a pan over high heat and add in sliced onions. Cook for approximately 10 minutes or until the onions are caramelized. Stir in vinegar and thyme and then remove from stove.
2. Mix together the broccoli and onion mixture in a bowl, adding salt and pepper if desired. Serve and eat salad as soon as possible.

Easy Butternut Squash Soup

Servings: 4 | Cooking: 1 Hour 45 min

Ingredients

- 1 small onion, chopped
- 4 cups chicken broth
- 1 butternut squash
- 3 tablespoons coconut oil
- Salt, to taste
- Nutmeg and pepper, to taste

Directions

1. Put oil and onions in a large pot and add onions.
2. Sauté for about 3 minutes and add chicken broth and butternut squash.
3. Simmer for about 1 hour on medium heat and transfer into an immersion blender.
4. Pulse until smooth and season with salt, pepper and nutmeg.
5. Return to the pot and cook for about 30 minutes.
6. Dish out and serve hot.

Nutrition: Calories: 149 Carbs: 6.6g Fats: 11.6g
Proteins: 5.4g Sodium: 765mg Sugar: 2.2g

Mediterranean Veggie Bowl

Preparation: 10 min | Cooking: 20 min | Servings: 4

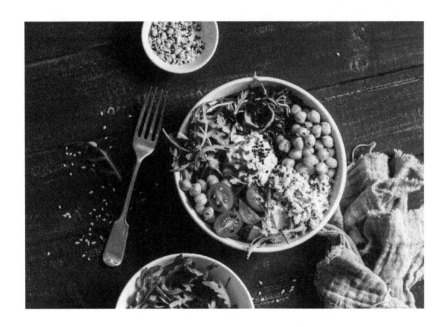

Ingredients

- 1 cup quinoa, rinsed
- 1½ teaspoons salt, divided
- 2 cups cherry tomatoes, cut in half
- 1 large bell pepper, cucumber
- 1 cup Kalamata olives

Directions

1. Using medium pot over medium heat, boil 2 cups of water. Add the bulgur (or quinoa) and 1 teaspoon of salt. Close and cook for 18 min.
2. To arrange the veggies in your 4 bowls, visually divide each bowl into 5 sections. Place the cooked bulgur in one section. Follow with the tomatoes, bell pepper, cucumbers, and olives.
3. Scourge ½ cup of lemon juice, olive oil, remaining ½ teaspoon salt, and black pepper.
4. Evenly spoon the dressing over the 4 bowls.
5. Serve.

Nutrition: 772 Calories: 6g Protein: 41g Carbohydrates

Baba Ganoush

Servings: 2 Tablespoons | Cooking: 50 min

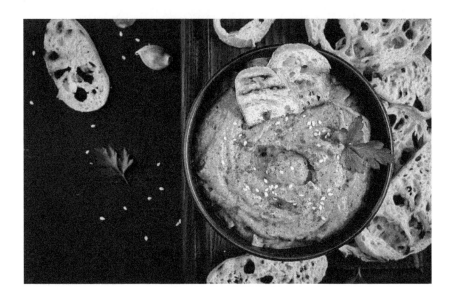

Ingredients

- 2 large eggplants
- 4 TB. extra-virgin olive oil
- 1 large white onion, chopped
- 1 TB. minced garlic
- 3 TB. fresh lemon juice
- 1 tsp. salt
- 1/2 tsp. ground black pepper

- 1/2 medium red bell pepper, ribs and seeds removed, and finely diced
- 1/2 medium green bell pepper, ribs and seeds removed, and finely diced
- 3 TB. fresh parsley, finely chopped
- 1/2 tsp. cayenne
- 3 medium radishes, finely diced
- 3 whole green onions, finely chopped

Directions

1. Preheat a grill top or a grill to medium-low heat.
2. Place eggplants on the grill, and roast on all sides for 40 minutes, turning every 5 minutes. Immediately place eggplants on a plate, cover with plastic wrap, let cool for 15 minutes.
3. Remove eggplant stems, and peel off as much skin as possible. (It's okay if it doesn't all come off.)
4. In a food processor fitted with a chopping blade, pulse eggplant 7 times. Transfer eggplant to a medium bowl.
5. In a medium saucepan over low heat, heat 2 tablespoons extra-virgin olive oil. Add white

onion, and sauté, stirring occasionally, for 10 minutes. Add onions to eggplant.

6. Add garlic, lemon juice, salt, black pepper, red bell pepper, green bell pepper, and parsley to eggplant, and stir well.

7. Spread baba ganoush on a serving plate, and drizzle remaining 2 tablespoons extra-virgin olive oil over top. Sprinkle with cayenne, radishes, and green onions.

8. Serve cold or at room temperature.

Leek And Potato Soup

Servings: 8 | Cooking: 1 Hour

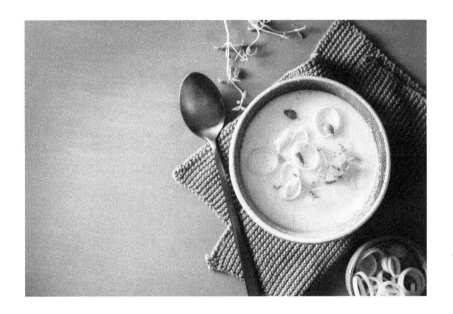

Ingredients

- 3 tablespoons olive oil
- 3 leeks, sliced
- 4 garlic cloves, chopped
- 6 potatoes, peeled and cubed
- 2 cups vegetable stock
- 2 cups water
- 1 thyme sprig
- 1 rosemary sprig

- Salt and pepper to taste

Directions

1. Heat the oil in a soup pot and stir in the leeks. Cook for 15 minutes until slightly caramelized.
2. Add the garlic and cook for 2 more minutes.
3. Add the rest of the ingredients and season with salt and pepper.
4. Cook on low heat for 20 minutes then remove the herb sprigs and puree the soup with an immersion blender.
5. Serve the soup fresh.

Nutrition: Calories:179 Fat:5.5g Protein:3.4g Carbohydrates:30.6g

Mast-o Khiar (Aka Persian Yogurt And Cucumbers)

Servings: 8 | Cooking: 10 min

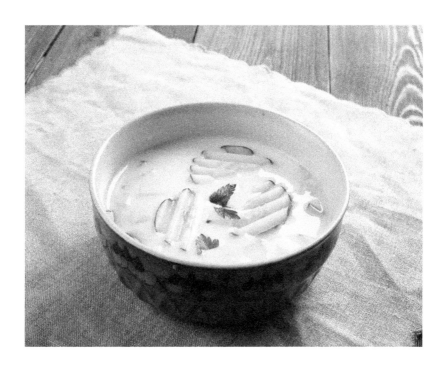

Ingredients

- 4 cup yogurt, plain Greek
- 2 teaspoon mint, dried
- 2 teaspoon dill, dried
- 1/4 teaspoon black pepper, ground
- 1/2 teaspoon salt

- 1 1/2 cup Persian cucumbers, diced

Directions

1. Combine all the ingredients in a medium-sized bowl.

Nutrition:62 cal., 4 g total fat (0.8 g sat. fat), 0 mg chol., 1 mg sodium, 81 mg pot., 7.2 g total carbs., 1.3 g fiber, 5.5 g sugar, 0.8 g protein, 0% vitamin A, 0% vitamin C, 1% calcium, and 3% iron.

Homemade Greek Yogurt

Servings: ½ Cup | Cooking: 20 min

Ingredients

- 1 gal. whole milk
- 2 cups plain Greek yogurt

Directions

1. In a large pot over medium-low heat, bring whole milk to a simmer until a froth starts to form on the surface. If you have a thermometer, bring the milk to 185°F.
2. Remove from heat, and let milk cool to lukewarm, or 110°F.
3. Pour all but about 2 cups milk into a large plastic container.
4. Pour remaining 2 cups milk into a smaller bowl. Add Greek yogurt, and stir until well combined.
5. Slowly pour milk and yogurt mixture into the large bowl of milk, and stir well.
6. Cover the bowl with a lid, and set aside where it won't be disturbed. Cover it with a towel, and let it sit overnight.

7. The next morning, gently transfer the bowl to the refrigerator. Chill for at least 1 day.
8. The next day, gently pour off clear liquid that's formed on top of yogurt, leaving just a little liquid remaining.
9. Serve, or store in the refrigerator for up to 2 weeks.

Curried Chicken, Chickpeas And Raita Salad

Servings: 8 | Cooking: 15 min

Ingredients

- 1 cup red grapes, halved
- 3-4 cups rotisserie chicken, meat coarsely shredded
- 2 tbsp cilantro
- 1 cup plain yogurt
- 2 medium tomatoes, chopped
- 1 tsp ground cumin
- 1 tbsp curry powder
- 2 tbsp olive oil
- 1 tbsp minced peeled ginger
- 1 tbsp minced garlic
- 1 medium onion, chopped
- ¼ tsp cayenne
- ½ tsp turmeric
- 1 tsp ground cumin
- 1 19-oz can chickpeas, rinsed, drained and patted dry

- 1 tbsp olive oil
- ½ cup sliced and toasted almonds
- 2 tbsp chopped mint
- 2 cups cucumber, peeled, cored and chopped
- 1 cup plain yogurt

Directions

1. To make the chicken salad, on medium low fire, place a medium nonstick saucepan and heat oil.
2. Sauté ginger, garlic and onion for 5 minutes or until softened while stirring occasionally.
3. Add 1 ½ tsp salt, cumin and curry. Sauté for two minutes.
4. Increase fire to medium high and add tomatoes. Stirring frequently, cook for 5 minutes.
5. Pour sauce into a bowl, mix in chicken, cilantro and yogurt. Stir to combine and let it stand to cool to room temperature.
6. To make the chickpeas, on a nonstick fry pan, heat oil for 3 minutes.
7. Add chickpeas and cook for a minute while stirring frequently.

8. Add ¼ tsp salt, cayenne, turmeric and cumin. Stir to mix well and cook for two minutes or until sauce is dried.

9. Transfer to a bowl and let it cool to room temperature.

10.   To make the raita, mix ½ tsp salt, mint, cucumber and yogurt. Stir thoroughly to combine and dissolve salt.

11. To assemble, in four 16-oz lidded jars or bowls layer the following: curried chicken, raita, chickpeas and garnish with almonds.

12. You can make this recipe one day ahead and refrigerate for 6 hours before serving.

Nutrition: Calories per serving: 381; Protein: 36.1g; Carbs: 27.4g; Fat: 15.5g

Chapter 7: Dessert Recipes

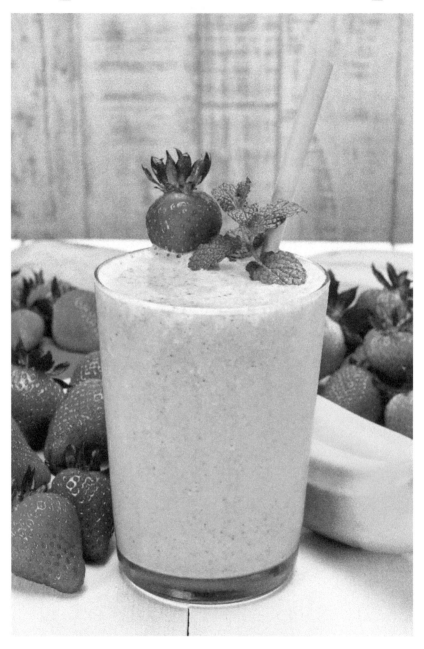

Yogurt Panna Cotta With Fresh Berries

Servings: 6 | Cooking: 1 Hour

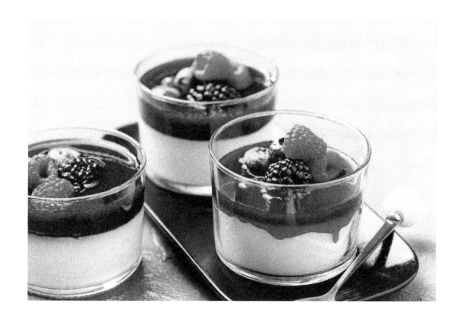

Ingredients

- 2 cups Greek yogurt
- 1 cup milk
- 1 cup heavy cream
- 2 teaspoons gelatin powder
- 4 tablespoons cold water
- 4 tablespoons honey
- 1 teaspoon vanilla extract

- 1 teaspoon lemon zest
- 1 pinch salt
- 2 cups mixed berries for serving

Directions

1. Combine the milk and cream in a saucepan and heat them up.
2. Bloom the gelatin in cold water for 10 minutes.
3. Remove the milk off heat and stir in the gelatin until dissolved.
4. Add the vanilla, lemon zest and salt and allow to cool down.
5. Stir in the yogurt then pour the mixture into serving glasses.
6. When set, top with fresh berries and serve.

Nutrition: Calories:219 Fat:9.7g Protein:10.8g Carbohydrates:22.6g

Flourless Chocolate Cake

Servings: 8 | Cooking: 1 Hour

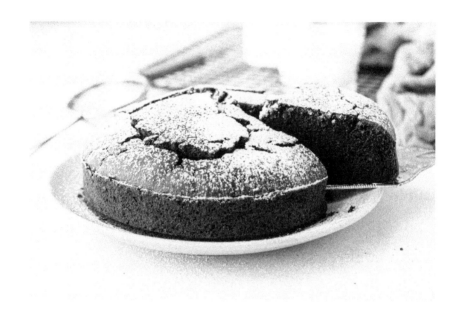

Ingredients

- 8 oz. dark chocolate, chopped
- 4 oz. butter, cubed
- 6 eggs, separated
- 1 teaspoon vanilla extract
- 1 pinch salt
- 4 tablespoons white sugar
- Berries for serving

Directions

1. Combine the chocolate and butter in a heatproof bowl and melt them together until smooth.
2. When smooth, remove off heat and place aside.
3. Separate the eggs.
4. Mix the egg yolks with the chocolate mixture.
5. Whip the egg whites with a pinch of salt until puffed up. Add the sugar and mix for a few more minutes until glossy and stiff.
6. Fold the meringue into the chocolate mixture then pour the batter in a 9-inch round cake pan lined with baking paper.
7. Bake in the preheated oven at 350F for 25 minutes.
8. Serve the cake chilled.

Nutrition: Calories:324 Fat:23.2g Protein:6.4g Carbohydrates:23.2g

Strawberry And Avocado Medley

Servings: 4 | Cooking: 5 min

Ingredients

- 2 cups strawberry, halved
- 1 avocado, pitted and sliced
- 2 tablespoons slivered almonds

Directions

1. Place all Ingredients: in a mixing bowl.
2. Toss to combine.
3. Allow to chill in the fridge before serving.

Nutrition: Calories per serving: 107; Carbs: 9.9g; Protein: 1.6g; Fat: 7.8g

Creamy Mint Strawberry Mix

Servings: 6 | Cooking: 30 min

Ingredients

- Cooking: spray
- ¼ cup stevia
- 1 and ½ cup almond flour
- 1 teaspoon baking powder
- 1 cup almond milk
- 1 egg, whisked
- 2 cups strawberries, sliced
- 1 tablespoon mint, chopped
- 1 teaspoon lime zest, grated
- ½ cup whipping cream

Directions

1. In a bowl, combine the almond with the strawberries, mint and the other ingredients except the cooking spray and whisk well.
2. Grease 6 ramekins with the cooking spray, pour the strawberry mix inside, introduce in the oven and bake at 350 degrees F for 30 minutes.
3. Cool down and serve.

Nutrition: calories 200; fat 6.3; fiber 2; carbs 6.5; protein 8

Watermelon Ice Cream

Servings: 2 | Cooking: 5 min

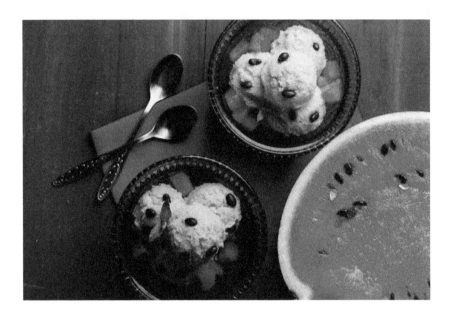

Ingredients

- 8 oz watermelon
- 1 tablespoon gelatin powder

Directions

1. Make the juice from the watermelon with the help of the fruit juicer.

2. Combine together 5 tablespoons of watermelon juice and 1 tablespoon of gelatin powder. Stir it and leave for 5 minutes.
3. Then preheat the watermelon juice until warm, add gelatin mixture and heat it up over the medium heat until gelatin is dissolved.
4. Then remove the liquid from the heat and pout it in the silicone molds.
5. Freeze the jelly for 30 minutes in the freezer or for 4 hours in the fridge.

Nutrition: calories 46; fat 0.2; fiber 0.4; carbs 8.5; protein 3.7

CPSIA information can be obtained
at www.ICGtesting.com
Printed in the USA
BVHW010550260621
610374BV00006BA/862